Published By Robert Corbin

@ Leah Myers

Plant Paradox Diet: Healthy and Easy Lectin Free

Recipes to Know About Plant Paradox Diet

All Right RESERVED

ISBN 978-1-7385954-3-3

TABLE OF CONTENTS

Avocado Salad And Cilantro-Pesto Chicken 1

Arugula Chicken Salad With Lemon Vinaigrette 4

Breakfast Tortilla 7

Zucchini Frittata 9

Peach Pancakes 12

Egg And Arugula 15

Ginger Carrot Soup 17

Green Pea Soup 18

Tasty Breakfast Hash 20

Breakfast Food Scramble 23

Chili Soup 24

Clear Onion Japanese Soup 26

Oats With All The Fuss 28

Black Bean And Sweet Potato Chili 31

Cabbage-Kale Sauté With Salmon And Avocado 35

Roasted Broccoli With Cauliflower "Rice" And Sautéed Onions 37

- Half tsp. of salt

- Half bell pepper (green, chopped)

- 4 zucchinis (cut in slices of half-inch)

- 4 tbsps. of parmesan cheese

Directions:
1. Start by preheating your oven at 160/175 degrees Celsius.
2. Take a large skillet and combine olive oil, water, green pepper, salt, garlic cloves, and zucchini.
3. Simmer the mixture until the zucchini is soft— Cook for seven minutes.
4. Drain the water and remove the garlic; add mushroom, onion, and butter.
5. Keep cooking until the onion turns transparent. Add the eggs and keep stirring.
6. Add pepper and salt for seasoning. Cook until the eggs are firm.

Zucchini Frittata

Ingredients:

- 3 garlic cloves (peeled)

- 2 onion (diced)

- Six mushrooms (chopped)

- 2 tbsp. of butter

- Five eggs

- Pepper and salt (to taste)

- 2 and a half cup of mozzarella cheese (shredded)

- 2 cup of water

- 4 tbsps. of olive oil

3. Spread the mixture of beans on half of the egg and flip 2 side for making the shape of a half-circle.
4. Cook until the eggs set properly.
5. Spread mayonnaise on the tortillas.
6. Cut the cooked eggs into 5 equal pieces. Place each piece of eggs on the tortillas. Top with lettuce.
7. Roll the tortillas. Serve hot.

Breakfast Tortilla

Ingredients:

- 2 tbsp. of mayonnaise

- 5 tortillas (flour)

- 2 and a half cup of lettuce (shredded)

- 3 tbsps. of beans (refried)

- 4 tbsps. of salsa

- 4 large eggs (beaten)

Directions:
1. Combine salsa and beans in a small bowl.
2. Take an iron skillet and heat oil in it. Add the eggs and let the bottom set—Cook for 2 minute.

lemon juice tablespoon with the olive oil and salt in a jar and shake until is homogeneous.
6. Add to the arugula and mushrooms.
7. Top with the chicken and pour some lemon zest.

- 2 tablespoons of lemon juice

- Sea salt to taste

Salad

- 1 1/2 cups chopped arugula

- Pan fried mushrooms

Directions:
1. Heat the avocado oil in a small pan on high heat.
2. Place the chicken strips in the pan and pour the lemon juice and salt.
3. Fry the chicken strips for 2 minutes; turn them and fry for another 2 minutes, until they're completely cooked.
4. Remove and save.
5. For the dressing, put 1 tablespoon of lemon juice over the avocado, and the bind the other

Arugula Chicken Salad With Lemon Vinaigrette

Ingredients:

Chicken

- 4 ounces of skinless, b2less chicken breast, cut into equal strips
- 1 tablespoon of lemon juice
- Zest of 1/2 lemon (optional)
- 1/4 teaspoon of iodized sea salt
- 1 tablespoon avocado oil

Dressing

- 1/2 diced avocado
- 2 tablespoons extra-virgin olive oil

6. For the dressing, put 1 tablespoon of lemon juice over the avocado, and the bind the other lemon juice tablespoon with the olive oil and salt in a jar and shake until is homogeneous.

- 1 1/2 cups chopped romaine lettuce
- 1/4 teaspoon iodized sea salt
- 2 cups of chopped cilantro
- 1/4 cup of extra-virgin olive oil
- 2 tablespoons of lemon juice

Directions:
1. Heat the avocado oil in a small pan on high heat.
2. Place the chicken strips in the pan and pour the lemon juice and salt.
3. Fry the chicken strips for 2 minutes; turn them and fry for another 2 minutes, until they're completely cooked.
4. Remove and save.
5. For the Pesto, all you need to do is put the ingredients in a mixer and blend them until they are all smooth.

Avocado Salad And Cilantro-Pesto Chicken

Ingredients:

Chicken

- 1/4 teaspoon of iodized sea salt
- 1 tablespoon avocado oil
- 4 ounces of skinless, b2less chicken breast, cut into equal strips
- 1 tablespoon of lemon juice

Pesto

- 1/2 diced avocado
- 2 tablespoons extra-virgin olive oil
- 2 tablespoons of lemon juice
- Sea salt to taste

Stuffed Mushrooms 124

Red Cabbage And Leek Casserole 126

Baked Kale Chips 129

Fruit Salad 131

Lentil Dal 133

Savory Waffles 136

Chocolate Waffles 137

Ginger, Blueberry Smoothie 139

Matka Smoothie Bowl 140

Mac And Cheeze With A Vegan Twist 142

Stuffed Sweet Potato 146

- Cranberry-Orange Muffin 80
- Garlic Bread And Veggie Delight 82
- Spinach Parmesan Balls 85
- Portobello Pizza 87
- Swedish Meatballs 89
- Spinach, Mandarin, And Walnut Salad 93
- Arugula And Roasted Pear Salad 95
- Avocado Cups 97
- Banana Pancakes 99
- Black, Lemon Chicken Soup 101
- Green Probity Smoothie 104
- Spinach And Tofu Lasagne 106
- Vegetable Britani 109
- Cinnamon-Flaxseed Muffin In A Mug 113
- "Green" Egg-Sausage Muffins 115
- Cinnamon And Flaxseed Muffin 118
- Sausage Muffins 120
- Cheese Garlic Bread 122

Roasted Broccoli With Cauliflower "Rice" And Pan-Fried Onions 40

Cabbage-Kale Sauté With Salmon And Avocado 43

Oatmeal And Strawberry Smoothie 45

Buffalo Cauliflower 46

Sweet Potato And Onion Patties 49

Sweet Potato Baked With Garlic And Kale 51

Quinoa Salad 53

Kale Blueberry Salad 56

Sweet Omelet 58

Australian Breakfast Omelet 60

Vegan Cauliflower Curry Soup 62

Mushroom Soup 64

Bean Veggie Burgers 66

Curried Chickpea And Broccoli Salad 70

Coconut-Almond Flour Muffin In A Mug 74

Cranberry-Orange Muffins 76

Coconut And Almond Flour Muffin 78

7. Add mozzarella cheese from the top.
8. Bake in the oven for ten minutes.
9. Remove the frittata from the oven and add parmesan cheese from the top.
10. Place under the broiler for about five minutes.
11. Cut the frittata in wedges and serve warm.

Peach Pancakes

Ingredients:

- Coconut flour, ¼ cup

- Tapioca, 1/4 cup

- Coconut oil, melted, 2 tablespoon

- Cassava flour, 1/4cup

- Seasalt, 1 teaspoon

- Baking soda, ¼ teaspoon

- Baking powder, 1/2 teaspoon

- 2 peaches, ripe. Peeled and sliced into thin slices

- Vanilla extract, 1 teaspoon

- 2 large eggs

- Monk fruit or stevia, 1 teaspoon

- Kefir or coconut yogurt, 5 ounces

- Cinnamon sprinkled over the peaches

Directions:
1. Prepare the oven by preheating to a temperature of 350 degrees and prepare a pie tray or pan with butter.
2. Using a lg bowl, add eggs, sweetener, kefir or coconut yogurt, and vanilla extract.
3. When adding these items into the bowl, gradually pour the coconut oil and whisk it continuously, to avoid the oil from sticking or becoming solid.
4. This is especially a concern if the room temperature is a bit cooler than usual.
5. Combine the cassava flour, coconut flour, sea salt, tapioca flour, baking soda, and baking

powder, using a med bowl, and blend well, then gently combine with the wet ingredients, a little at a time, until a smooth batter is formed.
6. Pour the batter into a pie pan and place the peach slices on top of the batter, then sprinkle with cinnamon evenly.
7. Cinnamon can also be sprinkled or coated over the peaches while mixing ingredients.
8. Cook for 30 min, then test with a toothpick to ensure it comes out clean, which means the pie-pancake is ready.
9. Serve with additional peach slices and whipped cream (coconut or dairy), and cinnamon.

Egg And Arugula

Ingredients:

- Sea salt, 1/2 teaspoon

- Fresh Arugula, 2 cups (chopped)

- 3 eggs

- Olive oil, 3 tablespoons, divided

- Balsamic vinegar, 2 tablespoons

Directions:
1. Using med heat and a lg skillet warm olive oil.
2. Using a sm bowl, whisk the balsamic vinegar, and sea salt together until well combined.
3. In a second bowl, whisk the eggs and add any desired spices, such as black pepper, paprika, etc. until blended.

4. Pour the eggs to scramble in the skillet, mixing evenly until they are well cooked.
5. Remove to a medium bowl, then mix the chopped arugula and drizzle the dressing over the dish to serve

Ginger Carrot Soup

Ingredients:

- 1 teaspoon of black pepper
- Dried or fresh parsley, for garnish
- 1 cup of coconut milk
- ½ cup of vegan sour cream
- 2 diced onions
- 5 cups of vegetable broth
- 3-4 cups of carrots, sliced
- 2 teaspoons of ground ginger (fresh)

Directions:

1. Cook the onions, carrots, and olive oil in a cooking pot that is large in size for about eight minutes in medium-heat setting, or until soft.

Green Pea Soup

Ingredients:

- 3 cups of vegetable broth

- 1 teaspoon of dill (fresh or dried)

- 1 teaspoon of tarragon

- 1 teaspoon of black pepper

- 1 bag of frozen peas

- 2 tablespoons of olive oil

- 1 onion, chopped

Directions:

1. Use a large-sized pot to warm the olive oil in a stove temperature set in medium-heat.
2. Add the onion, simmering for a couple of minutes.
3. Pour the broth and spices (tarragon, dill, and black pepper) and continue to cook, then increase the heat so that it begins to boil.
4. Lower the heat and add in the peas and cook on low-medium for about 10-15 minutes until peas are tender, then remove and chill. Use a food processor to pulse the soup batch by batch. Serve hot or cold.
5. This recipe makes 4-6 servings and takes about 30 minutes.
6. Add a dollop of coconut yogurt or sour cream on top of the soup when serving.

Tasty Breakfast Hash

Ingredients:

- 1 ½ lbs. grass-fed b2less chicken breasts, cubed
- 2 tablespoons olive oil, divided
- 1 tablespoon thyme, fresh chopped
- 2 tablespoons fresh lime juice
- 1 cup scallion, chopped
- 1 cup homemade chicken broth
- 1 tablespoon oregano, fresh chopped
- 4 garlic cloves, minced
- 1 medium white onion, chopped

- 2 celery sticks, chopped

- Salt and black pepper to taste

- 2 large sweet potatoes, cubed, peeled

Directions:
1. Add 1 tablespoon of oil into pan over medium heat and cook the chicken sprinkle with salt and pepper for about 5-minutes.
2. Transfer the chicken to a bowl.
3. With the same pan heat remaining oil over medium heat and sauté celery and onion for about 4 minutes.
4. Add in the garlic and herbs and sauté for about 1 minute.
5. Add the sweet potato and cook for 10 minutes.
6. Add the chicken broth and cook for an additional 10 minutes.

7. Add in the cooked chicken and scallion and cook for 5 minutes.
8. Stir in the lime juice, salt and serve.

Breakfast Food Scramble

Ingredients:

- 1 teaspoon garlic powder
- 2 cups kale, fresh, trimmed and chopped
- 2 tablespoons olive oil
- 4 fresh organic eggs
- Black pepper and salt to taste

Directions:
1. In a mixing bowl, add eggs and beat well. Set aside.
2. In a skillet, heat the oil over medium heat and cook the kale for 2 minutes.
3. Add eggs and remaining ingredients and cook for 4 minutes stirring often.
4. Serve hot and enjoy!

Chili Soup

Ingredients:

- ½ teaspoon olive oil

- 1 teaspoon sea salt

- ½ pound ground beef

- , Medium onion, roughly chopped

- C spoon ground canned pepper

- Water cup water

- ½ cup dairy cherry tomatoes

- On Spoon Garlic Powder

- 1 clove of garlic, crushed

- 1 teaspoon onion powder

- 1 tbsp chili powder

- 24 ounces can crush tomatoes

- Powder Tbsp Cumin Powder

Directions:
1. Fry onion, garlic and ground beef in a pan over medium heat.
2. Then, add fresh tomatoes, can tomatoes, and other spices.
3. Leave to boil over medium to low heat for 15-20 minutes.

Clear Onion Japanese Soup

Ingredients:

- salt and pepper to taste

- 1 carrot, diced

- 1 celery stalk, diced

- 1 handful chopped crust,

- 1 fist button mushroom, finely chopped

- 1 clove of garlic, minced

- 4 cups water or vegetable broth

- 1 medium sized onion, diced

- Soy sauce to taste

- Srirakha to taste.

Directions:

1. Over a medium heat, add some oil and fry the onion in a medium size pot and fry until slightly brown.
2. Then, add garlic, celery, carrots, and vegetable broth or water.
3. Bring to a boil, then simmer for 15-20 minutes.
4. Season with salt, pepper and other seasonings to taste.
5. Wash vegetables with water or broth, then add scallions and mushrooms before serving

Oats With All The Fuss

Ingredients:

Oats

- 1 ½ cups plant-based milk (of your choosing)
- ½ tbsp flaxseed (ground)
- 2 ½ tsp cinnamon
- 1 cup oats (steel cut rolled oats)
- 2 cups boiling water
- ½ tsp salt

Toppings

- 1 banana (small)
- ½ cup halved strawberries
- 2 tbsp dates (chopped)

- 1 tbsp cacao nibs (optional)

- 2 tbsp maple syrup

- 2 tbsp peanut butter (organic and sugar and salt-free)

Directions:
1. To create the warm morning oats it is quite quick and simple.
2. The toppings are completely up to and you should find the perfect combination for your taste buds.
3. Boil the water and milk (of your choice) in a medium pot.
4. Leave the heat at a low to medium heat before placing the oats, salt, and cinnamon in and giving it a good stir.
5. Add the flaxseed after about 3 minutes of cooking and continue the cooking for another 5 minutes.

6. Keep stirring quite often to avoid the gooey oats from sticking to the pot.
7. This recipe doesn't have to be exact and if you need more water, add it, or if you prefer less liquid, don't add in too much.
8. While the oats are softening up in the water, get your toppings ready by chopping, dicing, or slicing.
9. Once the oats are cooked, soft but not mushy, place them in a large bowl, slightly heat up the peanut butter in the microwave to a pourable state, and continue on with the assembling.
10. Drizzle the smooth, runny nut butter over the oats, and sprinkle the fruits in lines across the bowl (if you want that Integra shot), and add over any chopped nuts if you wish.
11. It is now ready for you to enjoy, you want to eat it warm so not too many photos!

Black Bean And Sweet Potato Chili

Ingredients:

- 2 cups vegetable broth

- 2 cups of water

- 1 cup dried quinoa

- 1 small lime (juiced)

- ½ small lemon (juiced)

- 1 small green chili

- 1 large avocado

- 2 tsp cumin

- 2 tsp chili paste

- 2 tsp smoked paprika

- 2 tsp ground coriander

- A dash of pepper

- 4 medium sweet potatoes (scrubbed and diced)

- 1 large yellow onion

- 4 cloves garlic (minced)

- 14 oz can of black beans

- 12 oz can crushed tomatoes

Directions:

1. Your first order of business is to chop and dice all your veggies. You will want to dice the potatoes into smallish cubes, roughly 1-inch, the onions and chili should be sliced, and lastly, mince the garlic.
2. Use a large pot to sweat the onions on a high heat with 1 tbsp of water before adding the

garlic and chili for 1 minute and then the sweet potatoes for another minute or 3.

3. Once the veggies are sizzling pour in the canned tomatoes, prepared vegetable broth, and can of beans. Lower that heat down to a gentle simmer and stir the delicious contents of the pot to let the flavors cook together. Toss in all the herbs and spices before giving it another big stir.

4. Leave the pot to do its work for 30 minutes, don't forget to give the chili a good stir occasionally to blend those sauces and veggies.

5. In the meantime cook up the quinoa by rinsing it well. Then place it in a pot, big enough to handle the amount of quinoa doubled, with boiling water. Once the water reaches a very fast boil, turn that heat down to medium for a gentle simmer to arise and

leave it to cook, with the lid on, for up to 20 minutes when all the water has dried up.
6. Once dried up, turn the heat off and leave the lid on for a 5 minute steam.
7. Pour it into a bowl and give it a good fluff up with a fork, add the lime juice before giving it another shake up.
8. The avocado must be prepared by mashing it in a bowl, adding a touch of pepper and the lemon juice, leaving those flavors to meet each other.
9. Once the potatoes are tender enough to be easily pierced with a fork, turn the stove off leaving the chili to thicken slightly before pouring over a bed of fluffy quinoa and topping with creamy mashed avocado.

.

Cabbage-Kale Sauté With Salmon And Avocado

Ingredients:

- 1½ cups finely sliced green cabbage

- ½ red onion, thinly sliced

- 3 ounces wild-caught Alaska salmon

- ½ avocado, diced

- 3 tablespoons freshly squeezed lemon juice

- 4 pinches sea salt, preferably iodized

- 3 tablespoons avocado oil

Directions:

1. Toss the diced avocado in 1 tablespoon of the lemon juice and season with a pinch of salt. Set aside.

2. Heat a skillet over medium heat. When it is hot, add 2 tablespoons of the avocado oil and the cabbage and onion.
3. Sauté until tender, about 10 minutes, stirring occasionally.
4. Season with 2 more pinches of salt.
5. Using a slotted spatula, remove from the skillet and set aside.
6. Add the remaining 1 tablespoon avocado oil to the skillet, raise the heat to high, and add the remaining 2 tablespoons lemon juice and the salmon.
7. Sear the salmon, flipping after 3 minutes, until cooked through, about 6 minutes total.
8. Season with the remaining pinch salt.
9. To serve, top the sautéed cabbage and onions with the salmon and avocado.

Roasted Broccoli With Cauliflower "Rice" And Sautéed Onions

Ingredients:

Cauliflower "rice"

- 1 tablespoon freshly squeezed lemon juice

- ¼ teaspoon curry powder

- 1 pinch sea salt, preferably iodized

- ½ head medium cauliflower, riced (see headnote)

- 1 tablespoon avocado oil

Broccoli

- 1½ tablespoons avocado oil

- 1 pinch sea salt, preferably iodized

- 1½ cups cut-up broccoli florets

Curried onions

- ½ red onion, thinly sliced
- Pinch sea salt, preferably iodized
- ½ tablespoon avocado oil

Directions:

1. Heat the oven to 375°F, Sauté the cauliflower in a medium skillet with 1 tablespoon of the avocado oil, the lemon juice, curry powder, and a pinch of salt until tender, 3 to 5 minutes.
2. Do not let it get mushy by overcooking.
3. Transfer the cauliflower "rice" to a plate and keep warm.
4. Wipe the skillet clean with a paper towel.
5. Put the broccoli in a Pyrex dish with 1 tablespoon of the avocado oil.

6. Roast in the oven for 15 minutes, stirring twice, until tender. Season with a pinch of salt.
7. Reheat the skillet over medium heat. When it is hot, add the remaining ½ tablespoon avocado oil and the sliced onion and sauté until tender, stirring frequently, for about 5 minutes. Season with a pinch of salt.
8. To serve, place the cauliflower "rice" on a plate and top with the broccoli and sautéed onions.

Roasted Broccoli With Cauliflower "Rice" And Pan-Fried Onions

Ingredients:

For the Cauliflower "Rice"

- 1 tablespoon of lemon juice

- A pinch of sea salt

- 1/4 teaspoon of curry

- Half a medium head of a riced cauliflower

- 1 tablespoon of avocado oil

For the Broccoli

- 1 1/2 cups of cut broccoli buds

- 1 tablespoon of avocado oil

- A pinch of sea salt

For the Sautéed onions

- 1/2 tablespoon avocado oil

- A pinch of salt

- Diced onions

Directions:
1. Preheat the oven to 325°F.
2. Sauté the cauliflower in a medium pan with 1 tablespoon of avocado oil, and the lemon juice, curry powder, and a pinch of salt until it is tender, about 3 to 5 minutes.
3. Pass it to a plate and keep it warm. Wipe the pan clean.
4. Put the broccoli in an oven safe plate with 1 tablespoon of the oil.
5. Roast it for 15 minutes, blending it twice, until it is tender.
6. Add a tad of salt.

7. Reheat the frying pan and when it is hot, add the remaining tablespoon avocado oil, the diced onion and a pinch of salt.
8. Fry until tender, stirring often, for about 5 minutes.
9. To serve, place the cauliflower "rice" on a plate and on top of it, the broccoli and stir-fried onions.

Cabbage-Kale Sauté With Salmon And Avocado

Ingredients:

- 3 tablespoons of avocado oil
- 1 1/2 cups of thinly sliced cabbage (green, bok choi or your preferred cabbage)
- 1/2 red onion, thinly sliced
- 3 ounces of wild-caught salmon
- 1/2 diced avocado
- 4 pinches of iodized sea salt
- 3 tablespoons of lemon juice

Directions:
1. Mix diced avocado with 1 tablespoon of lemon juice and a drop of salt.
2. Heat a pan to medium heat.

3. Then, add 2 tablespoons of oil and all of the cabbage and onion.
4. Fry for 10 minutes or until it's tender, stirring once in a while, and add 3 pinches of salt.
5. Remove.
6. Now add the last tablespoon of oil to the skillet, raise the heat and put in the salmon.
7. Add the rest of the lemon juice and a pinch of salt.
8. Sear it 3 minutes each side and you can serve.

Oatmeal And Strawberry Smoothie

Ingredients:

- 5teen strawberries (frozen)
- 2 banana (cut in chunks)
- 3 tsps. of agave nectar
- 2 cup of almond milk
- Half cup of rolled oats
- Half tsp. of vanilla extract

Directions:
1. Add almond milk, strawberries, oats, agave nectar, banana, and vanilla extract in a food processor. Keep blending until smooth.
2. Serve with pieces of strawberry from the top.

Buffalo Cauliflower

Ingredients:

- 2 large egg

- Six cups of cauliflower florets

- 3 cups of garlic croutons

- 2-5th cup of parmesan cheese (grated)

- 2 serving of cooking spray

- Half cup of buffalo sauce

- 4 tbsps. of mayonnaise

For the dipping sauce:

- 2-5th cup of each

- Sour cream

- Blue cheese salad dressing

- 2 tsp. of black pepper (ground)

Directions:
1. Start by preheating your oven to 230 degrees Celsius.
2. Use a cooking spray for greasing a baking tray.
3. Combine mayonnaise, buffalo sauce, and egg in a bowl.
4. Toss the florets of cauliflower in the mixture of sauce and coat properly.
5. Spread the tossed florets on the baking tray.
6. Add the croutons on a blender and pulse them into crumbs.
7. Add the cheese and pulse again.
8. Spread the mixture of cheese and croutons over the florets of cauliflower.
9. Bake for fifteen minutes until tender and browned.
10. Allow the florets to sit for five minutes.

11. Mix all the ingredients for the dipping sauce.
12. Serve cauliflower florets with dip sauce by the side.

Sweet Potato And Onion Patties

Ingredients:

- Sea salt / ground black pepper, as desired

- Paprika, ½ tsp

- Chili-pepper, ½ teaspoon

- Olive oil for cooking

- 1 large or 2 med sweet potatoes

- 1 small onion, white or yellow, diced finely

- 1 large or 2 small or medium eggs

Directions:

1. To prepare the sweet potatoes, scrub, peel and slice them into halves, thirds, or sizes that are comfortable to shred through a grate.

2. Using a large grater, shred all the sweet potato and set aside.
3. Peel the onion and slice in half and shred or finely dice to mix with the sweet potato.
4. Mix these 3 ingredients well with a fork, then add in the eggs, whisking and blending evenly.
5. Add in the sea salt, black pepper, paprika, and chili pepper, to create the patty batter.
6. Over med heat and a lg skillet warm olive oil.
7. As the skillet is in the process of warming up, form 2-inch or 3-inch sized patties to fry on both sides of the skillet.
8. If desired, add a light sprinkle of sea salt and/or the spices and seasoning of your choice.
9. Cook on each side for about 2 minutes, or until the result is golden in color.
10. Serve immediately garnished with sliced parsley, coriander, and/or sour cream.

Sweet Potato Baked With Garlic And Kale

Ingredients:

- Kale (any variety, finely sliced with stems removed), 1 cup

- Sea salt

- 2 crushed garlic cloves

- Sweet potatoes (1 small or medium)

- Olive oil

Directions:
1. Peel, wash, and scrub the sweet potato and make a few slices into the top, or poke with a fork.
2. Wrap the potatoes in tin foil and poke with the fork a couple of times.

3. Set oven to 350 degrees, once preheated, add the dish for approximately 45-60 min or until the sweet potatoes are tender and flaky inside.
4. They can be baked directly in the rack in the oven or a pan.
5. As the sweet potatoes bake, prepare a skillet with 2 tablespoon of olive oil.
6. Toss in the crushed garlic cloves, sliced kale, and sea salt.
7. Saute on medium until the kale is crispy (or almost crispy). If the kale is d2 before the sweet potatoes, turn off the stovetop and cover with a lid until they are ready.
8. Serve the sweet potatoes with a drizzle of olive oil and top with the garlic and kale mix to serve.

Quinoa Salad

Ingredients:

- 1 red bell pepper, diced

- ½ cup of dried cranberries and/or blueberries

- ½ cups of mixed sunflower seeds, pumpkin seeds, crushed walnuts, pecans, and other nuts

- ½ cups of fresh parsley, dill, mint, basil, and/or cilantro

- 1 cup of uncooked quinoa

- 1 small or medium cucumber (sliced, about 2 cup)

- 2 cups of water

- 2 cups of bok choy

For the dressing:

- 3 tablespoons of olive oil

- Dash of black pepper

- 2 tablespoons of lemon juice (freshly squeezed)

- Dash of sea salt

- 1 teaspoon of maple syrup or low carb sweetener

- 2 tablespoons of apple cider vinegar

Directions:
1. In preparing the dressing, you need to put together first and mix all the ingredients for the dressing in a small mixing container before setting it aside.
2. Combine the salad ingredients and toss evenly, then serve with the vinaigrette.

3. This dish makes about 4-6 servings and takes about 15-20 minutes to prepare.

Kale Blueberry Salad

Ingredients:

- 1 cup of fresh blueberries
- ½ cups of sliced almonds
- 1 bunch of kale (stems removed, sliced or shredded)

For the dressing:

- 1 teaspoon of maple syrup
- 2 tablespoons of lime or lemon juice
- 2 teaspoons of olive oil

Directions:
1. Mix the 4 ingredients for the vinaigrette in a mixing dish that is small in size before setting

it aside. In a larger bowl, combine the sliced kale, and toss in the fresh blueberries.
2. Serve sprinkled with the vinaigrette and topped with sliced almonds.

Sweet Omelet

Ingredients:

- ½ large green apple, cored and thinly sliced
- 2 teaspoons olive oil, divided
- ¼ teaspoon nutmeg
- Pinch of salt
- 1/8 teaspoon organic vanilla extract
- 2 large organic eggs
- ¼ teaspoon ground cinnamon

Directions:
1. In a non-stick frying pan, heat the 1 teaspoon of oil over medium-low heat and cook apple slices, nutmeg, and cinnamon for about 5

minutes, turning once halfway through the cook time.
2. In a mixing bowl, add eggs, vanilla and salt beat until fluffy.
3. Add remaining oil into the pan and allow it to melt completely.
4. Add the egg mixture over apple slices evenly, cook for 4 minutes.
5. Carefully, turn the pan over a serving plate and then fold the omelet and serve hot.

Australian Breakfast Omelet

Ingredients:

- Salt and freshly ground black pepper to taste

- 4 large organic eggs

- 2 small beets, peeled and spiralized with Blade C

- 2 tablespoons olive oil, divided

- 1 teaspoon chives, fresh minced

- 1 small avocado, peeled, pitted and cubed into small pieces

Directions:

1. Using a large pan, heat 1 tablespoon olive oil over medium heat and cook the beet noodles for about 7 minutes.
2. Remove from heat and set aside.

3. Add to your mixing bowl, salt, pepper and eggs then beat well.
4. Heat the remaining oil in large frying pan over medium heat.
5. Add your egg mixture to your pan and spread the eggs over pan using a wooden spoon.
6. Cook the egg mixture for 12 minutes.
7. Place the beets and avocado over the eggs.
8. Carefully, fold the omelet over the beet noodles and avocado and cook for 2 minutes.
9. Cut the omelet into 3 portions and serve with the chives for garnish.

Vegan Cauliflower Curry Soup

Ingredients:

- Toasted macadamia nuts, sliced for garnish
- C teaspoon ground cumin
- Sea salt to taste
- ½ head cut cauliflower into bite-sized pieces
- 1 cup full-fat coconut milk
- Sliced Sitaphal for garnish
- 1 tbsp Extra-Virgin Olive Oil
- 1 teaspoon fresh ginger, finely chopped
- 1 teaspoon curry powder

- 4 cups homemade vegetable broth or chicken broth

- Ch onion, chopped

- 1 garlic clove, minced meat

Directions:
1. Heat extra virgin olive oil in a saucepan.
2. Add in garlic, cauliflower, onion, spices and ginger.
3. Stir the cauliflower until it is brown and the onion is translucent.
4. Then, add vegetable or chicken broth, sea salt and coconut milk.
5. Reduce heat and cook until tender.
6. Blend the mixture, and adjust the spice to your taste.
7. Then, serve the soup and garnish with macadamia nuts, cilantro, and coconut yogurt.

Mushroom Soup

Ingredients:

- ¼ cup raw walnuts, or almond butter or hemp seed hearts

- ¼ teaspoon iodized sea salt

- Spoon Truffle Oil (optional)

- 1/8 teaspoon black pepper cracked.

- 2 tablespoons chopped red onion

- 1 fresh oregano sprig

- 1 tablespoon mushroom stem

- ½ cup water

Directions:

1. Cut the mushrooms in half and set aside.

2. Add leftover mushrooms, walnuts, salt, onion, parsley, black pepper and water to the food processor.
3. Pulse ingredients for 25–30 seconds, then mix for 1 minute.
4. Inspect the mixture for temperature, it should be hot.
5. However, if you like it hot, you can either mix on high for 1 minute or put the ingredients in a saucepan for too long and simmer for a few minutes.
6. Take out of heat and pour the soup into the soup bowl.
7. The texture should be gravy-like and thick.
8. Then, garnish your soup with sliced mushrooms and drizzle with truffle oil.

Bean Veggie Burgers

Ingredients:

Black bean patty

- ½ cup green onion
- ½ cup walnuts
- 1 tsp smoked paprika
- 1 tsp chili powder
- 1 tbsp soy sauce (low sodium)
- 2 tsp maple syrup
- 15 oz can of black beans (rinsed and drained, or use 1 ½ cups cooked beans)
- ½ cup rolled oats
- ½ cup breadcrumbs

- 3 cloves garlic

- 1 small shallot (or ½ large white onion)

Toppings

- 4 slices of tomato

- ½ avocado sliced

- 2 whole wheat hamburger buns

- 2 leaves of lettuce

Directions:
1. These bean patties can be made by hand if you prefer a chunkier texture or in a food processor for a smoother patty.
2. By hand, finely dice or mince the garlic, shallots, and green onion. The walnuts should be chopped finely as well.
3. Drain the beans and blot them dry before pouring them into a large bowl. Add in the

minced veggies, the oats, and the breadcrumbs. Using a fork or potato masher, create a chunky batter before sprinkling over the spices, maple syrup, and soy sauce.

4. Again you will need to mix these together, using your hands will create a good base for your burger.

5. If you are using a food processor add all the above ingredients (excluding ½ the beans) before blending them to desired consistency. Add the last beans at the end to create a chunky texture.

6. When everything is well blended, place the bowl in a cool spot to let it gel together for a minimum of 10 minutes.

7. This mixture can be kept for 24 hours in the fridge if you would like to prepare it ahead of time.

8. Once the flavors are well acquainted, split the mix into 3 or 5 portions, first rolling them into

tasty balls and then squishing them flat to create discs.
9. Heat up a pan with 2 tbsp water to fry up the beany goodness, 7 minutes per side over a medium heat should let them cook through nicely.
10. They can also be baked in the oven at 350°F for 20 minutes, flipping them over halfway through.
11. Toast the hamburger buns in the oven if desired and assemble your burger with the remaining toppings.

Curried Chickpea And Broccoli Salad

Ingredients:

Salad

- ½ cup dried cranberries
- ½ cup sliced almonds (or chopped)
- ½ cup fresh cilantro
- 1 tbsp chopped chives
- 1 head of broccoli (chopped up finely)
- 15 oz can of chickpeas (drained)
- 1 cup sliced carrots

Dressing

- 2 tsp maple syrup
- 1 garlic clove (minced)

- ½ tsp turmeric
- 1 tsp mild curry powder
- ½ tsp grated ginger
- 1 tsp garlic powder
- ¼ tsp salt
- 1 tsp onion powder
- ¼ cup tahini
- 4 tbsp water (lukewarm will work well)
- ½ small lemon (juiced)
- Black pepper to your liking

Directions:

1. *Once the oven is warmed up to* 400°F pop in the chickpeas laid out on a baking tray with a touch of salt and pepper.

2. Let them roast to a slight crisp for 15-20 minutes.
3. Next get going with the dressing to give the flavors time to meld and strengthen, offering your taste buds a more tantalizing experience.
4. Create this zingy delight by throwing all the dressing parts into a mixing bowl, except the water, and bring those flavors together with a good whisk.
5. Slowly add in the water while still stirring since you don't want it to become too watery.
6. Stop pouring the water when it reaches your desired thinness, you want it to pour easily.
7. Use a heat-friendly bowl to microwave the broccoli with a small amount of water for 4 minutes.
8. The broccoli should be cut into small bite-sized pieces for the perfect mouthfuls of zesty salad.

9. Once heated, drain the water and add the broccoli to your favorite salad bowl as a perfect salad base.
10. Mix in the remaining of the salad bits (without the almond flakes) and do the great salad toss.
11. Drown the salad with the zingy dressing making sure every inch is nicely coated before throwing in the almond flakes and roasted chickpeas before giving 2 final shake.
12. The curried salad will only increase in flavor if left in the fridge for a few days and it can be kept for up to 5 days if you can wait that long after smelling the fresh curry flavors.

Coconut-Almond Flour Muffin In A Mug

Ingredients:

- ½ teaspoon aluminum-free baking powder

- Pinch sea salt, preferably iodized

- 1 packet stevia, or 2 teaspoons Just Like Sugar

- 1 tablespoon water

- 1 large pastured or omega-3 egg, lightly beaten

- 1 tablespoon extra-virgin coconut oil, melted

- 1 tablespoon extra-virgin olive oil or macadamia nut oil

- 1 tablespoon coconut flour

- 1 tablespoon almond flour

Directions:

1. Place the ingredients in an 8- to 12-ounce microwave-safe mug, mixing well with a fork or spatula. Be sure to scrape the bottom and sides. Let it sit for a few seconds.
2. Microwave on high for 1 minute plus 25 to 30 seconds.
3. Using a pot holder, remove the mug from the microwave and invert, shaking out the muffin. Let cool for a couple of minutes before eating.

Cranberry-Orange Muffins

Ingredients:

- ¼ cup extra-virgin coconut oil, melted

- ¼ cup Just Like Sugar or xylitol

- 3 large pastured or omega-3 eggs

- 1 tablespoon orange zest

- ¼ cup coconut flour

- ¼ teaspoon sea salt, preferably iodized

- ¼ teaspoon baking soda

- ½ cup dried, unsweetened cranberries

Directions:

1. Heat the oven to 350°F. Line a standard 6-cup muffin tin with paper liners.

2. Place the coconut flour, salt, and baking soda in a food processor fitted with an S-blade.
3. Add the coconut oil, Just Like Sugar, eggs, and orange zest.
4. Pulse until blended. Remove the processor blade and stir in the cranberries by hand.
5. Scoop the batter into the muffin tins, filling to just beneath the rim.
6. Bake for 20 minutes. Let cool on a rack for 15 minutes before serving.

Coconut And Almond Flour Muffin

Ingredients:

- 1 tablespoon of almond flour
- 1 pinch of iodized sea salt
- 1 tablespoon of water
- 1 large lightly beaten egg
- 1 tablespoon of melted coconut oil
- 1 tablespoon of olive or macadamia nut oil
- 1 pack of stevia
- 1/2 teaspoon of baking powder
- 1 tablespoon of coconut flour

Directions:

1. Place all of the ingredients in a mug that's somewhere between 8 to 12 ounces and mix them well with a spatula scraping the bottom and sides of the mug.
2. Let it stand and microwave it for 1 minute.
3. Let it stand again and microwave them for another 30 seconds.
4. Remove the mug and invert it using a pot holder.
5. Let it stand for a couple of minutes before you eat it.

Cranberry-Orange Muffin

Ingredients:

- 1/4 teaspoon of sea salt
- 1/4 cup of melted coconut oil
- 1/4 cup of xylitol
- 3 large eggs
- 1 tablespoon of orange zest
- 1/2 cup of unsweetened cranberries
- 1/4 cup of coconut flour
- 1/4 teaspoon of baking soda

Directions:
1. Preheat the oven to 350°F.
2. Line a 6-cup muffin tin with paper liners.

3. Then, put the flour and baking soda in a food processor.
4. Add the oil, the xylitol, eggs, and zest.
5. Process it until it's blended.
6. Remove the blade and mix in the cranberries with a spatula.
7. Scoop the mix into the tins and bake for 20 minutes.
8. Let them cool for 15 minutes before you eat them.

Garlic Bread And Veggie Delight

Ingredients:

- 2 eggplant (cubed)
- 2 zucchini (cubed)
- 2 tomato (chopped)
- 2 tsp. of salt
- 3 tsps. of each
- Basil (minced)
- Oregano (minced)
- 2 cup of olive oil
- 2 garlic clove (chopped)
- 2 baguette

- 5 tsps. of garlic powder

- Six tsps. of butter

Directions:

1. Take a large skillet and add olive oil to it. Add garlic and fry for 3 minutes until browned.
2. Add the zucchini and eggplant to the skillet and cook for five minutes.
3. Make sure that the eggplant is tender and brown.
4. Add the chunks of tomato and combine the veggies; add basil, oregano, and salt.
5. Cook for 3 minutes and remove from heat.
6. Preheat oven 140/165 degrees Celsius.
7. Slice the baguette into 2-inch slices, approximately twelve slices.
8. Add butter and garlic powder on the bread slices and place them on the oven rack.
9. Heat the bread for five minutes.
10. Arrange the heated bread slices on a plate.

11. Top the slices with vegetables. Serve immediately.

Spinach Parmesan Balls

Ingredients:

- Half cup of butter (melted)
- 5 green onions (chopped)
- 5 eggs (beaten)
- Pepper and salt (for seasoning)
- Twenty ounces of frozen spinach (chopped)
- 3 cups of bread crumbs
- 2 cup of parmesan cheese (grated)

Directions:
1. Start by preheating your oven at 175 degrees Celsius.
2. Take a bowl and combine spinach, bread crumbs, cheese, green onions, butter, pepper,

salt, and eggs. Make balls of 2-inch size from the prepared mixture.
3. Arrange the spinach balls on a baking tray. Bake for fifteen minutes until browned.
4. Serve hot.

Portobello Pizza

Ingredients:

- Shredded mozzarella cheese, 1 cup

- Pepperoni or prosciutto slices

- Olive oil

- Sea salt and black pepper

- Portobello mushroom caps

- Basil pesto, 1-2 teaspoons

Directions:

1. If desired, grill or roast the Portobello mushroom caps for 2-3 minutes, then top with a drizzle of olive oil, shredded mozzarella cheese, pepperoni or prosciutto slices, basil pesto, and top with black pepper, sea salt

and/or other spices and seasoning, as preferred.
2. Set oven to 350 degrees, once preheated add pizza fr approximately 20 min, until crust is golden and serve.

Swedish Meatballs

Ingredients:

- Onion powder, 1 teaspoon

- Mustard powder, ½ teaspoon

- White or yellow onion, finely diced, ¼ cup

- Mushrooms, 4 large, diced or minced

- Ground black pepper, ¼ teaspoon

- Parsley, chopped finely, fresh or dried, ¼ cup

- 1 egg

- 1 lb of ground beef

- Sea salt, 1 teaspoon

- Almond flour, 3 teaspoons

To make the sauce:

- Balsamic vinegar, 1 tsp

- Garlic powder, 1 tsp

- Sour cream or coconut cream (dairy-free sour cream alternative), ¾ cup

- Parsley, finely chopped or diced, 2 tablespoons

- Sea salt and black pepper to taste

- ¼ ground mustard powder

- Fish sauce, 1 teaspoon

- Coconut oil or butter, 1 tablespoon (olive oil can also be used)

- White onion, sliced, ½ cup

- Mushrooms, 4 large, sliced

- Beef broth or stock, 2 cups

Directions:
1. To prepare this recipe, preheat the oven to a temperature of 425 degrees and use a silic2 mat or tin foil to line a cookie or baking sheet.
2. Combine the ground beef, mushrooms, minced onions, eggs, parsley, spices, and almond flour in a large bowl.
3. When the ingredients are well mixed, form into balls that are roughly 1-2 inches in diameter.
4. Make sure each of the portions are equal in size, then place on the tray.
5. Bake for approximately 10-12 min, then flip meatballs and continue cooking for 9-10 min, until they are brown and cooked thoroughly.
6. As the meatballs bake, the sauce can be prepared.

7. Over med-hi heat use a large skillet to warm coconut oil or butter, then toss in the mushrooms and onion.
8. Saute these ingredients for 4-5 minutes, the mushrooms and onions should become tender.
9. Pour in the beef stock or broth and stir for a minute, then add in the spices, fish sauce, and balsamic vinegar to cook on medium for another 5 minutes.
10. Place the meatballs into the sauce and cook on low, simmering for about 7-8 minutes or until the sauce is lighter and reduced in volume.
11. Take the skillet off of the burner and stir in the sour cream (or coconut cream), then top with parsley.

12. Add a bit of sea salt and ground black pepper, then serve with salad, noodles, or a side dish of your choice.

Spinach, Mandarin, And Walnut Salad

Ingredients:

- 3-4 mandarins, peeled and pieces (slices) removed

- 1 cup of coarsely chopped walnuts

- ½ cup of shredded carrots

- 1 bunch of spinach, washed and drained

For the dressing:

- 3 teaspoons of orange juice (freshly squeezed)

- 1 teaspoon of maple syrup

- 2 teaspoons of olive oil

Directions:

1. Mix the ingredients for the salad dressing in a small bowl and set aside.
2. In a larger bowl, add the fresh spinach (washed and drained in a colander), and toss in the shredded carrots, walnuts, and mandarin slices.
3. Serve with dressing. This recipe makes approximately 4-5 servings and can be prepared within 15 minutes.

Arugula And Roasted Pear Salad

Ingredients:

- 2 cups of chopped arugula

- 1 roasted pear, sliced in half

- ½ cups chopped walnuts

- 1 cup of coarsely chopped pecans

For the dressing:

- 2 teaspoons of lime juice

- 2 teaspoons of olive oil

- 1 teaspoon of maple syrup

Directions:
1. To roast the pear, set the oven to 350, slice the pear in half, and place face down on a

baking sheet prepared with a parchment paper.
2. Bake for half an hour, then remove and cool for 10-15 minutes.
3. Mix the dressing ingredients together well, then set aside.
4. Combine all the salad items and blend evenly. Lightly coat with dressing and serve.

Avocado Cups

Ingredients:

- 1 tablespoon chives, fresh minced
- Salt and freshly ground black pepper to taste
- 4 organic eggs
- 2 ripe avocados, halved, pitted and scoop out about 2 tablespoons of flesh

Directions:
1. Preheat your oven to 425°Fahrenheit.
2. Arrange the avocado halves in a small baking dish, with the cut side facing upwards.
3. In a mixing bowl, break an egg then transfer it into an avocado half.
4. Repeat this step with the remaining eggs.

5. Carefully, place into your oven and bake for 20 minutes or until you have reached the desired d2ness reached.
6. Serve immediately, sprinkle with salt and pepper and chives

Banana Pancakes

Ingredients:

- 1 teaspoon apple cider vinegar
- ½ teaspoon ground cinnamon
- ¼ teaspoon organic baking powder
- ¼ cup coconut flour
- ½ teaspoon organic vanilla extract
- 2 teaspoons olive oil
- 1 tablespoon organic h2y
- 1 ripe banana, peeled and mashed
- 2 organic eggs
- ½ cup unsweetened almond milk

- Pinch of salt

Directions:
1. In a large mixing bowl, mix baking powder, flour, cinnamon, and salt.
2. In another bowl, add egg, banana, almond milk, h2y, vinegar, and vanilla, beat well until well combined.
3. Add the mixture into your flour mixture and mix well.
4. Grease a frying pan with olive oil and heat over medium heat.
5. Add the desired amount of mixture and cook for 3 minutes.
6. With a spatula, flip over the pancake and cook for 2 more minutes.
7. Repeat with remaining mixture and serve warm.

Black, Lemon Chicken Soup

Ingredients:

- Oon Spoon Dijon Mustard

- Half lemon juice

- Black pepper, fresh ground to taste

- 1 tablespoon fresh lemon juice

- 1 stalk celery, minced or chopped

- 1 bunch bananas, sliced into 1 inch pieces

- Freshly Permigiana Regigo, freshly grated (for service)

- 2 teaspoons extra-virgin olive oil

- 3 cloves garlic, minced

- Oon Spoon Balsamic Vinegar

- 3 cups homemade salt free chicken or vegetable stock

- ½ medium onion, finely cooked

- Sea salt to taste

- ½ cup cooked chicken, chopped or sliced.

Directions:
1. Over medium heat, heat extra-virgin olive oil in a large saucepan (crock-pot or Dutch oven).
2. Pour in garlic, onion, and celery, along with a small pinch of black pepper and sea salt.
3. Pan-fry until the celery is very tender, and the onions become translucent.
4. Pour with cubed or sliced chicken, kale, and djon mustard, lemon zest, and pan-fry for 3-5 minutes.

5. Pour in vegetable or chicken broth, lemon juice and balsamic vinegar, then reduce heat.
6. Cover the pot, warm for 20-25 minutes before serving.

Green Probity Smoothie

Ingredients:

- ¼ cup frozen mixed berries
- ¼ avocado, peeled and pitted
- ¼ cup coconut milk
- Ha Kombucha Tea
- 1 teaspoon chia seeds
- 1 fist baby spinach
- 1 teaspoon grass fed collagen

Directions:
1. In a food processor mix all the ingredients together with a discount for chia seeds.
2. After the ingredients are blended until smooth.

3. Then add in chia seeds, do some quick pulse to mix well.

Spinach And Tofu Lasagne

Ingredients:

- ¼ cup cashews
- ¼ cup of soy milk
- 2 tbsp lemon (juiced)
- 2 tbsp fresh basil (crushed)
- 32 oz can of crushed tomato
- ½ tsp onion powder
- 1 tsp dried herbs
- ½ tsp garlic powder
- 3 tbsp nutritional yeast
- ½ lb lasagna sheets (whole wheat)

- 8 oz block of firm tofu

- 8 oz block of soft tofu

- 20 oz frozen spinach

- 2 garlic cloves (minced)

Directions:

1. *Prepare your oven by switching it to 325°F to* let it heat up to cook this tasty lasagne.
2. The spinach should be placed in a tray to thaw while the cashews are left to soak in a bowl of water for at least 30 minutes.
3. Get rid of the excess water in the tofu by pressing the blocks with something heavy while the rest of the parts are heating up, soaking, or thawing.
4. Once your items are prepared, blend the tofu along with the garlic and cashews either in a food processor or a blender.

5. Create a ricotta cheese-like paste before throwing in the remaining ingredients (without the pasta sheets, canned tomatoes, and nutritional yeast).
6. Assemble the layers by creating a thin layer of the crushed tomatoes followed by a layer of pasta sheets, more sauce then the tofu mix, and repeat 4 times.
7. The top should have a layer of tomato sauce, with a dusting of creamy sauce and nutritional yeast to finish it off.
8. Let it bake and bubble away in the oven for 30 minutes. Allow the top layer of lasagna pieces that are peaking out to crisp up ever so slightly.

Vegetable Britani

Ingredients:

- 3 cloves garlic (chopped)
- 1 tbsp ginger
- 4 cups vegetable stock
- 1 tbsp chili powder
- 1 tbsp coriander
- 1 tbsp cumin
- ½ tsp turmeric
- ½ tsp cardamom
- ½ tsp salt
- ½ cup raisins

- 15 oz can of chickpeas (rinsed and drained)
- 2 cups brown basmati rice (rinsed)
- 1 cup bell pepper (sliced thinly)
- 1 cup zucchini (sliced thinly)
- ½ cup carrots (shredded)
- 1 large onion
- 1 bay leaf

Directions:

1. Firstly slice up your veggies, including the onions which should also be sliced thinly, and rinse your chickpeas and rice.
2. Splash a dash of oil, or water if you have reached your minimum oil use for the week, in a large wok or pan and heat it up high.
3. Sauté the onions on their own for 3 minutes before tossing in the rest of the veggies,

garlic, and ginger to sweat them all out. You can change up the veggie choices if you wish.
4. Let these all cook well together on medium heat for around 5 minutes.
5. Next, the spices and bay leaf need to be added, toast them up nicely in the mix for 2 minutes.
6. Take another minute to let the dry mix toast up once you have tossed in the rice. Then quickly pour in the stock and make sure everything is mixed together.
7. Push the heat up to high while pouring in the chickpeas and raisins until a fast simmer arises.
8. Once the bubbles begin, drop it down to low and let it cook away for 35 minutes.
9. If the water has dried up and the rice is not cooked yet, slowly add some more water or stock.

10. You want the water to have all dried up before removing it from the stove but only as long as the rice has cooked properly.
11. Serve and enjoy or store it away for another meal.

Cinnamon-Flaxseed Muffin In A Mug

Ingredients:

- 1 tablespoon extra-virgin coconut oil, melted
- 1 teaspoon aluminum-free baking powder
- 1 packet stevia
- ¼ cup ground flaxseed
- 1 teaspoon cinnamon
- 1 large pastured or omega-3 egg

Directions:
1. Place all the ingredients in an 8- to 12-ounce microwave-safe mug, and mix well with a fork or spatula.
2. Be sure to scrape the bottom and sides. Let it sit for a few seconds.
3. Microwave on high for 1 minute.

4. Check and cook for another 5 to 15 seconds if the muffin appears still wet in the center.
5. Using a pot holder, remove the mug from the microwave and invert, shaking out the muffin. Let cool for a couple of minutes before eating.

"Green" Egg-Sausage Muffins

Ingredients:

- 2 cloves garlic, peeled, or 1 teaspoon garlic powder

- 2 tablespoons Italian seasoning

- 2 tablespoons dried minced onion

- ½ teaspoon sea salt, preferably iodized

- ½ teaspoon cracked black pepper

- 1 pound Diestel Farms Turkey Italian Sausage or Turkey Chorizo

- One 10-ounce bag chopped organic frozen spinach (or chopped kale)

- 5 pastured or omega-3 eggs

- 2 tablespoons extra-virgin olive oil or perilla oil

Directions:
1. Heat the oven to 350°F. Line a standard-size 12-cup muffin tin with paper liners.
2. Crumble the sausage or chorizo and put in a non-Teflon frying pan.
3. Cook over medium-high heat, stirring frequently, until browned, about 8 to 10 minutes. Set aside.
4. With a sharp knife, poke small holes in the bag of spinach, put in a microwavable bowl, and place in the microwave on high for 3 minutes.
5. Cut a tiny edge off the corner of the bag, and squeeze as much water out of the bag as possible.
6. Place the drained spinach, eggs, olive oil, garlic, Italian seasoning, onion, salt, and pepper in a high-speed blender and

pulse/blend for about 1 minute, or until thoroughly mixed.
7. Transfer to a large bowl and stir in the sausage until well mixed.
8. Fill the muffin tins to just beneath the rim.
9. Bake for 30 to 35 minutes, until the tops start to brown.
10. Remove from the oven and let cool before removing individual muffins from the liner.

Cinnamon And Flaxseed Muffin

Ingredients:

- 1 teaspoon of baking powder

- 1 pack of stevia

- 1 tablespoon of coconut oil

- 1/4 cup of grounded flaxseed

- 1 teaspoon cinnamon

- 1 large pastured egg

Directions:

1. Put all of the ingredients in a mug that's somewhere between 8 to 12 ounces and mix them well with a spatula scraping the bottom and sides of the mug.
2. Let them sit for a few seconds, and then microwave on high temperature for 1 minute.

3. Let it stand for a few seconds and check if the muffin is still wet in the center if so, cook for another 15 seconds.
4. Remove the mug and invert it using a pot holder.
5. Let it stand for a couple of minutes before you eat it.

Sausage Muffins

Ingredients:

- 2 tablespoons of Italian seasoning

- 2 tablespoons onion powder

- 1/2 teaspoon of sea salt

- 1/2 teaspoon of cracked pepper

- 2 tablespoons extra-virgin olive oil

- 1 teaspoon of garlic powder

- 1 pound of Turkey Italian Sausage or Turkey Chorizo

- 2 10-ounce bag of chopped spinach or kale

- 5 pastured eggs

- 2 cloves peeled garlic

Directions:
1. Preheat the oven to 350°F.
2. Line a 6-cup muffin tin using paper liners.
3. Mash the sausage and put in on a frying pan and cook it on medium heat for 10 minutes.
4. Poke small holes in the spinach or kale bag, put in a bowl, and place in the microwave for 3 minutes.
5. Cut an edge off the bag's corner and squeeze the water out.
6. Place all the ingredients but the sausage in a blender and mix for about 1 minute.
7. Put it in a bowl and mix in the cooked sausage.
8. Scoop the mix into the tins and bake for 35 minutes and let it rest a bit before eating.

Cheese Garlic Bread

Ingredients:

- Thyme (dried)
- Garlic powder
- 2 tbsp. of parmesan cheese (grated)
- 2 loaf of French bread (halved)
- Half cup of butter (melted)
- 2 tsp. of garlic salt
- 2-5th tsp. of rosemary (dried)
- 2-eighth tsp. of each
- Basil (dried)

Directions:

1. Preheat oven at 150 degrees Celsius.

2. Mix garlic salt, butter, basil, rosemary, thyme, garlic powder, and cheese in a bowl.
3. Spread the butter mixture on the halves of the bread.
4. Add extra cheese from the top if you want to.
5. Place halves of bread on a baking tray. Bake for twelve minutes until browned.

Stuffed Mushrooms

Ingredients:

- 9 ounces of cream cheese (softened)
- 2-5th cup of parmesan cheese (grated)
- 2-5th tsp. of each
- Onion powder
- Black pepper (ground)
- 12 whole mushrooms
- 2 tbsp. of each
- Minced garlic
- Vegetable oil
- Cayenne powder (ground)

Directions:

1. Preheat the oven to 175 degrees Celsius.
2. Grease a baking tray with the help of cooking spray.
3. Clean the mushrooms using a damp kitchen towel; break the stems. Chop the mushroom stems finely.
4. Take a skillet and heat oil in it.
5. Add chopped stems of mushroom and garlic— Cook for five minutes.
6. Remove the skillet from heat and let it cool. Add the cream cheese, black pepper, parmesan cheese, cayenne powder, and onion powder. Mix well.
7. Use a small spoon for filling the mushroom caps with the mushroom stuffing.
8. Place the mushroom caps on the prepared baking tray.
9. Bake for twenty minutes until liquid forms under the mushroom caps.

Red Cabbage And Leek Casserole

Ingredients:

- Sea salt and ground black pepper to taste

- Fennel seeds, ½ teaspoon

- Fresh or dried dill, 1 teaspoon of dried, or a small handful of fresh and finely diced

- Olive oil for cooking, extra virgin oil is recommended

- Large or medium head of cabbage (red or green cabbage)

- 2 medium-sized leeks, washed and sliced (green onions can be used if leeks are not available)

Directions:

1. To prepare the cabbage, shred with a large grater by hand and into a large bowl.
2. The amount of cabbage may appear excessive at first, though once cooked, it will reduce in size.
3. Prepare the oven by preheating to a temperature of 400 degrees.
4. Slice the leeks finely and add them to the cabbage to distribute and blend evenly.
5. Add in the fennel seeds, dill, ground black pepper, and sea salt to mix. Line a casserole dish with parchment paper and lightly sprinkle with oil.
6. Once the ingredients in the bowl are well mixed, pour them into the casserole dish and drizzle the olive oil evenly over the ingredients.
7. Place the casserole dish into the oven to bake for 15 minutes on the middle rack of the oven.

8. If the vegetables are not softened enough, you may bake for another 15-20 minutes. Serve immediately as the main dish, or as a tasty side.
9. There are many variations to this dish, including adding sliced kale, shredded cauliflower or broccoli florets, and onions, if desired.
10. This is a dish that is experimented with and changed at your leisure, with a variety of vegetable blends and flavors.
11. Additional spices, such as chili powder, paprika, cumin, and many others, are also welcome to this dish and can a unique and satisfying twist to the flavor as well.

Baked Kale Chips

Ingredients:

- Kale -2 bundle

- Seasalt

- Olive oil

Directions:
1. This is a simple recipe that involves only 4 main ingredients and can be made within 15 minutes.
2. To prepare the kale, remove the stems and slice the leaves into bite-sized pieces.
3. Wash and dry thoroughly, then sprinkle on a lite coat of olive oil and put it on a lined tray, then sprinkle lightly with sea salt.
4. Coconut or avocado oil can be used if olive oil is not available.

5. Once you have preheated the oven tp 350 degrees cook for approximately 8 10 min.
6. Check the oven between 8 and 10 minutes to monitor the progress of the kale, making sure they are not overcooked or burnt.
7. If removed too early, the kale chips will be wet and undercooked, and if a minute too late, they may be burnt.
8. Knowing when to remove them from the oven may take 2 or 3 attempts if this is your first time making these chips.

Fruit Salad

Ingredients:

- 1 cup of sliced cantaloupe or h2ydew into cubes

- 1 cup of sliced watermelon

- ½ cup of sliced strawberries stems removed

- ½ cup of blueberries

- ½ cup of raspberries

- 1 cup of sliced pineapples

- 1 large apple, sliced (skin can be removed or left on)

- 1-2 mandarins, peeled and broken apart into slices/pieces or 2 large orange, sliced and skin removed

- 1 cup of grapes (seedless)

Directions:

1. This salad is easy to prepare and may include as little or as many of the fruits above (and more).
2. Wash, chop, and assemble all fruits and drain in a colander.
3. Serve with freshly squeezed lemon and garnish with fresh mint leaves.
4. The salad serves 4-6 and takes approximately 15-20 minutes to prepare.

Lentil Dal

Ingredients:

- 2 teaspoons of grated ginger (fresh is recommended)

- 1 small or medium tomato, diced

- 1 teaspoon of paprika

- ½ teaspoon of cardamom

- 1 teaspoon of turmeric

- 1 teaspoon of sea salt

- 1 teaspoon of lemon juice

- 1 teaspoon of chili powder (optional)

- 1 green chili pepper, diced (with stem removed)

- 1 cup of diced onion (white or yellow)

- 1 tablespoon of olive oil

- 2 teaspoons of cumin seeds

- 1 cup of red lentils

- 1 teaspoon of cinnamon

- 4 crushed garlic cloves

- 1 cup of chopped parsley or cilantro leaves

Directions:

1. If using dried lentils, rinse and bring to a boil in a saucepan covered in water, reduce, and cook on medium for 15-20 minutes.
2. While the lentils are cooking, let a skillet heat up before adding the olive oil, cumin, and cinnamon on medium for five minutes, then add in the garlic, onion, green chili, chili powder (optional ingredient), and ginger.

3. Simmer for another five or six minutes, then add the following items: salt, tomatoes, paprika, cardamom, and turmeric.
4. Continue to cook for another five minutes.
5. When the lentils are cooked, drain and stir in the skillet mixed with the lentils, combining evenly.
6. Add fresh lemon juice. Serve with cilantro or parsley leaves.

Savory Waffles

Ingredients:

- 1/2 teaspoon dried rosemary, crushed
- 1/8 teaspoon red pepper flakes, crushed
- 1 medium sweet potato, peeled, grated and squeezed
- Salt to taste

Directions:
1. Preheat the waffle iron and grease it.
2. In a bowl, add ingredients and mix well.
3. Add half of the mixture in preheated waffle iron and cook for 10 minutes.
4. Repeat with the remaining mixture.
5. Serve warm.

Chocolate Waffles

Ingredients:

For waffles:

- ¼ cup coconut flour

- ½ teaspoon baking soda

- ½ teaspoon organic vanilla extract

- ¼ cup 70% dark chocolate chips

- 1 cup blanched almond flour

- ¼ cup cacao powder

For sauce:

- 2 tablespoons coconut oil

- ¼ cup 70% dark chocolate chips

Directions:

1. Preheat the waffle iron and grease it.
2. In a mixing bowl, mix together cocoa powder, baking soda, flours, and salt.
3. In another bowl, add h2y, vanilla extract and eggs mix well.
4. Add the egg mixture into bowl with flour mixture and mix well.
5. Gently, fold in chocolate chips.
6. Add ¾ cup of mixture to waffle iron. Cook for 5 minutes.
7. Repeat with remaining mixture.
8. For the sauce, in a small pan, add coconut oil and chocolate chips over low heat and melt while stirring continuously.
9. Serve the waffles with the topping of chocolate sauce.

Ginger, Blueberry Smoothie

Ingredients:

- Stevia to taste
- CT Spoon MCT Oil
- ¼ tbsp collagen powder
- 12 blueberries
- Ut Cup Coconut Yogurt
- ½ cup 240 ml coconut milk mixed
- 2 slices ginger
- 1 slice apple

Directions:

1. Add all ingredients to a food processor and mix until smooth.

Matka Smoothie Bowl

Ingredients:

- 1 teaspoon greens powder (optional)
- Stevia to taste
- ½ teaspoon goji berries
- 1 teaspoon coconut flakes
- Ch Tbsp Chia Seeds
- Oon Spoon Matka Powder
- 6 oz Coconut Yoghurt or Greek Yoghurt
- C Tbsp cacao nibs

Directions:

1. Add the curd to the matka and mix. If you wish, add it to stevia to make it sweeter. Empty the mixed smoothie in a bowl.
2. Garnish with cacao nib, chia seeds, coconut flakes and goji berries.

Mac And Cheeze With A Vegan Twist

Ingredients:

- 1 tbsp white wine vinegar

- 2 tbsp nutritional yeast

- 1 tsp onion powder

- ½ tsp fresh thyme (finely chopped)

- ¼ tsp salt

- ¼ tsp black pepper

- 8 oz penne pasta (whole grain)

- 1 medium butternut squash

- 3 cups broccoli florets

- 4 cloves garlic (minced)

- 1 onion (chopped finely)

- 2 cups plant-based milk (unsweetened and unflavored will work well)

Directions:

1. Start off by cooking the pasta in a large pot of boiling water with the pinch of salt.
2. Go according to the package instructions, and then 5 minutes before the pasta has reached its al dente state, pop in the broccoli to boil away.
3. Now get on with steaming the squash; after you have peeled and deseeded it, put it into a steamer dish with water below the basket and bring the water to a boil on a high heat on top of the stove.
4. Let the squash steam away for 12 minutes.
5. The squash should be tender enough for a fork to easily pierce through it when it is ready.

6. On the other side of the stove get a pan going over medium heat with 2 tbsp of water.
7. The onion, garlic, and thyme should be cooked in this pan until the onion has softened up nicely.
8. This can take 10 minutes and you may need to add water as you go to stop the onions from sticking to the bottom of the pan.
9. Once this is cooked up and the squash is ready, transfer these to a blender (let it all cool down for 5 minutes first) then add in the milk, nutritional yeast, vinegar, salt, and pepper.
10. Flip the switch to blend them all up, to create a creamy and smooth sauce ready to cover your pasta.
11. Pour this into your pan used to cook the onion mix, and heat it up as you toss in the cooked pasta and broccoli.

12. Use small kitchen tongs to easily combine these all together so the sauce is covering every inch of pasta.

Stuffed Sweet Potato

Ingredients:

Potatoes

- 1 tsp lemon juice

- 2 tsp nutritional yeast

- 1 tsp onion powder

- 1 tsp pepper

- 2 large sweet potatoes

- 15 oz can of black beans (or 1 ½ cup of cooked beans)

- ½ a large avocado (more if you are bulking up)

- 1 tsp garlic powder

Salsa

- 2 limes (juiced)
- ½ tsp cumin
- 1 tsp maple syrup
- 4 large tomatoes
- ½ white onion
- 3 cloves garlic
- 1 jalapeño
- ½ cup cilantro

Directions:
1. The oven will need to be heated ahead of cooking so start it up to 450°F.
2. Once the oven is nice and toasty, lay the potatoes on a baking tray, poke them a few

times with a fork to create holes for the steam to escape and then leave them in the oven for 40 minutes.
3. While the sweet potato is dispensing aromas from the oven prepare your salsa by chopping up all the veggies.
4. Cut the onions and tomatoes into chunks, deseed the jalapeño and cut into chunks, and roughly slice up the garlic too.
5. Throw all the salsa ingredients into a blender and blitz it all up to a chunky consistency.
6. If you don't have a blender you can finely chop the veggies up by hand and then mix it all together to bring the flavors together.
7. Heat the beans up in a pan with a splash of water and spice with the onion and garlic powder.
8. Once the potatoes are steaming hot, make sure a fork can pierce through them easily, remove them and let them cool down slightly

before cutting them open down the middle. Cut them longways to ensure more space to fill them up.
9. Dust the inside with the nutritional yeast before spooning on the beans and then the salsa.
10. In a small bowl, mash the avocado and season with pepper and lemon juice.
11. Top the potatoes with the creamy avocado and you're good to go.

www.ingramcontent.com/pod-product-compliance
Lightning Source LLC
Chambersburg PA
CBHW071457080526
44587CB00014B/2138